What people are saying about Andrea Thatcher

"Andrea is one of the very best instructors. She is constantly seeking new knowledge to understand and to then pass on to others. Andrea is very genuine and professional when presenting. "
Shaun Harris, RMT, D.O.M.P. Candidate.

"Andrea Thatcher is tireless and relentless in her pursuit to help and inspire others. If there were more people like Andrea in the world, there would be a lot more happiness and a lot less dis-ease. I love having Andrea as a colleague in the health and fitness industry."
Dr. Greg Long, Chiropractor,
ProActive Health Chiropractic and Massage Performance Centre.

"I am writing to you today to express my sincere gratitude for what you have done for me. You have changed my life in many ways, as a teacher, a nutritionist, a mentor and a personal trainer. What I am most grateful for is the wealth of knowledge on nutrition that you have taught me. In past, I had always thought I was very knowledgeable when it came to nutrition but when you began to teach me natural nutrition, you opened my eyes to a new way of thinking and eating. At 57 I feel healthier, stronger and happier with myself than ever before.
Lil Foster – Retired Business Owner

"When I attended one of your Nutrition seminars for the first time, I was not disappointed! You taught in detail about how the actual nutrient content in food is altered and this has had a significant impact on the way I now prepare food for my family. I am very grateful to you for teaching this valuable information, which is contributing daily to the improvement of my own health, and the health of my family."
Karen Kildaw – Mom

"The information that you shared in your Natural Nutrition Workshop regarding flour and its effects on our digestive systems has

been extremely valuable to me. There are several instances of poor colon health in my extended family, and I had been afraid that I was doomed to the same fate. The difference in the dispositions of my children since reducing their wheat flour intake has been remarkable."
Trevor Brown

"Information on nutritional supplementation can be difficult to understand, and is often contradictory between sources. Andrea addressed supplementation, and it has completely revolutionized the way I take my supplements! She taught in detail regarding supplements taken in pill form, specifically regarding ingredients, manufacturing and absorption. We are a healthy, energetic family and we owe this to Andrea"
Karen Brown - Personal Trainer

"Andrea, I've been dealing with progressively worsening Psoriasis for several years. Based on your suggestions, I have taken processed foods (specifically sugar) out of my daily diet. After only a few weeks, I've noticed that my psoriasis has very noticeably decreased. I intend to continue to follow your good advice as the positive effects far outweigh the convenience of eating processed foods and sugars."
Leonard VandenBerg – Stone Mason

"Andrea, you have taught me that we don't need to diet in order to lose weight. We merely need to eliminate toxic food products, and note the difference in our mood, energy levels and waistlines.

If I can feel this good in only a few days, then I'm definitely going to keep this up! It's not radical in any way; it's simply a matter of ditching the junk and replacing it with real food. So simple."
Joey Saks, Personal Trainer

IN
ONE END
AND OUT
THE OTHER

An Intensive Guide To Everyday Nutrition

Andrea Thatcher,

Registered Holistic Nutritionist, (RHN)

www.AndreaThatcher.com

Published by Zana Books

Zana Books ISBN: 9-780988-1647-2-7

Visit ZanaBooks.com

Library and Archives Canada Cataloging in Publication

Thatcher, Andrea
In One End and Out the Other... An Intensive Guide To Everyday Nutrition

ISBN: 9-780988-1647-2-7

1. Health and Fitness I. Title.

HD57.7.S37 2012658.4'092C2012-906179-9

Printed in Canada

DEDICATION

This book is dedicated to each of those I have worked with, for without you, I would not have the opportunity to do what I love to do each day. Thank you for choosing to work with me and allowing me to live my passion of helping others live their personal best.

TABLE OF CONTENTS

The 80/20 Rule 11

Eating, Naturally...15

    Natural Nutrition...15

    Understanding Certified Organic Foods....................15

Nutrition - The Basics..25

Understanding Nutrients..31

Macronutrients 33

    Carbohydrates..33

    Protein 42

    Fat...48

    Water 53

Micronutrients 56

    Minerals..56

    Vitamins 56

What You Should Know About Calories...........................59

Understanding an Ingredient Label..................................64

Understanding Sugar and Sugar on Your Labels 69

    Hidden Sugars?..70

    The Harmful Kind of Sugars 73

    Healthier Sweetening Options 74

    Health Effects of Sugar 76

Weight Loss and Weight Gain..80

Eating and Exercising 85

Working towards a healthy diet 88

Eating Habits 100

Conclusion 101

Success Stories 102

Introduction

This book is about what it truly takes be healthy with natural nutrition. I've taken the most common questions I've been asked over the years and put them here with the answers as I see it.

It's time you heard the truth. You have been misled by the media, large corporations, and sales people looking to make a buck. Let's start by telling you that there is no magic pill, lotion, potion, quick fix, or secret food that is going to improve your health. Your health will improve when you make small changes to your current way of eating, and consistently choose natural foods that will improve your health. I know it would be so great if we could just take a pill, or a shake, or pre-packaged wonder food and improve our health, lose weight, and have unlimited energy. It's just not how it works.

Repetitive marketing message on tv and magazines offering sensational products in a box or a can or a carton have chiselled away at our common sense and over time have convinced us that lies are truth, and we have lost sight of the simplicity needed to improve and maintain our health with food.

I'm done hearing and seeing this garbage. I have decided I won't sit back and watch my loved ones destroy their health and appearance and lose track of what was important. I wrote this book to take you, and your loved ones back to the basics. I'm going to help you weed your way through the crap that's out there and make simple decisions based on common sense and nature. You can begin to make small changes to your food choices right away, and you can completely change how you feel. You know that you can get the body, the energy and the health levels you want, you just need to know how. This book will help you make better nutrition choices, and when you do, you'll feel better for it.

How do I know that you can improve your health and your quality of life through natural nutrition? Well... 8 years ago, I suffered from terrible depression and anxiety, I was overweight, tired all the time, couldn't sleep, couldn't stay alert at work and felt like crap every day. I was introduced to natural nutrition, and I'm offering you living proof that it works. I made my health a priority, and I followed the principles of healthy eating. Within a year, I was no longer medicated for depression or anxiety, I had lost the 30 pounds, and I am so thankful I now sleep peacefully through the night with unlimited energy during the day. I am happy!

In addition to personal experience I am also schooled in Natural Nutrition. I have worked as a leader in the fitness industry, teaching and certifying thousands of Personal Trainers and Nutrition and Wellness Specialists with canfitpro. I have counselled thousands to make better decisions to improve the quality of their lives, and from this experience I have taken what works and what doesn't.
This book is about what matters, and what works—the basics; the way we were designed to live. No fluff, no lose 30 pounds in 30 days promises, no magic. Just the basics—Simple.

I hope this book will shake your current way of thinking into a new way of thinking. I hope it will trigger your curiosity to learn more, and bring a greater state of health into your life. It's time to create new nutritional behaviours and habits and create a new way of eating: For your health, for your body, for you.

Meet Andrea

Andrea Thatcher is considered an expert and one of the most respected professionals in her industry for her extensive knowledge, integrity and her ability to create results in the lives of those she works with.

Andrea is dedicated to the success of all individuals in reaching their personal best, through healthy fitness, nutrition and wellness. Andrea is a passionate woman, providing educational workshops, seminars and one on one coaching for individuals, to ensure all goals are reached successfully.

In addition to being a Registered Holistic Nutritionist, (RHN) and being trained as a Holistic Lifestyle Coach, she has worked as a fitness consultant for more than 18 years, and is further trained as a Reiki Master/Teacher. Andrea is also a leading instructor and examiner for *canfitpro*, certifying thousands of Personal Trainers and Nutrition and Wellness Specialists across Canada. Andrea was awarded **2010 PRO TRAINER of the year.**

Andrea has created and implemented programs for The St. Joe's Hospital department of Eating Disorders, Mental Health Unit, and worked side by side with psychologists and dietitians. She has created an International Certification program for Weight Management, to name a few of her accomplishments.

Andrea is a gifted presenter and coach, teaching her audience and clients in a professional and zealous fashion. She has the ability to translate difficult information and tailor it to the learning needs of each she works with. Known for her boundless energy and bubbling enthusiasm, her students, clients and attendees find her motivating, inspiring and fun to work with.

THE 80/20 RULE

Before we begin, I want to share THE most important tool for your success. During this book I will share with you the best and healthiest food and nutrition choices. With that being said, it is important that you apply the '80/20 rule' to everything I say. Here's the lowdown on the 80/20 rule:

Cast your mind over the last ten years and ask yourself how many times you swore this was it - your *final* attempt at dieting, getting on track, giving up vices, and so on. If you failed each time, ask yourself why. The answer is likely that you were seeking perfection. No one is perfect, and striving for perfection will lead to failure – every time.

Coming oh-so-close to perfection is definitely *not* outright failure. So consider eating the 80/20 way, and free yourself from the belief that your only options are perfection or failure.

The 80/20 method is simple. Essentially, 80% of the time you are making healthy food choices that feed your PHYSICAL body. And

20% of the time you are making any choice you want that feeds your SOCIAL, SPIRITUAL and EMOTIONAL body.

It is absolutely ridiculous to think that when you eat a salad your body loses weight, but when you eat a cookie, it goes straight to your thighs. Sorry folks, your bodies just aren't that refined. Your can easily work through 20% of your diet coming from less than perfectly healthy foods. What this means for you:

If you eat 4 times a day, 7 days a week, that's 28 meals. Accordingly, approximately 5 meals a week can consist of whatever you choose.

Another way of looking at it: 6 days a week you eat only healthy foods, and on the 7th day you eat whatever you want.

If you're a person who needs visual cues, think of it this way: ensure that 80% of your plate is healthy food and 20% of it is whatever you want.

If you're a long-term planner, here's yet another way to consider it: there are 365 days each year. That's 73 days of eating whatever you want!

The key to success here is to eat these meals GUILT FREE. Feeling guilty after eating causes more damage to your body than the less-than-perfectly-healthy food ever could.

Now that we've given ourselves permission to occasionally enjoy less-than-perfect foods, let's examine the most common reasons why we eat them at all:

Convenience: Fast food allows us to cram more and more into our already crowded schedules. We can eat on the run and feel like we're maintaining productivity.

Boredom: Eating is a great (and mindless!) way to pass the time. Especially when there's a TV involved.

Habit: We eat out of habit at certain times and in certain places. For example, wouldn't it feel weird to go to the movies and NOT eat popcorn?

Comfort: Food can provide tremendous emotional comfort when we are sad or lonely.

There is _absolutely_ room in a healthy diet for convenience, boredom, habit and comfort! Simply be aware of what you are eating, and strive to make healthy choices 80% of the time.

Choose what you can sustain - realistically - when life happens. Perfection sucks.(And it's boring!!!)

NOTES:

Eating, Naturally

Natural Nutrition

Natural Nutrition means eating foods that come from the earth, in their natural state, that have not been processed. Fresh fruits, fresh vegetables, raw nuts and seeds, whole eggs, raw milk, beans and lentils, whole grains such as quinoa and wild rice, and meat such as wild game, beef, chicken, turkey, pork, fish or seafood are examples of whole foods that come from the earth. Basically, if it grows, it's natural.

Understanding Certified Organic Foods

'Certified organic foods' refer to foods which are grown and/or produced without being exposed to any kind of fungicide, herbicide, pesticide, and/or chemical fertilizer. Organic farming relies on getting its needs met through what Mother Nature has to offer, and is not only good for our health, but helps preserve the environment as well.

The 'organic' certification is given only three years after the farm in question starts practising the guidelines set-forth by the Organic committee. This waiting period gives the soil the time to eliminate and digest any kind of chemical residue that could be present in the soil from previous years. Bear in mind that foods, during this waiting period, can still be labelled organic, even though the soil may not be fully rid of chemicals, and this is why it's always better to buy Certified Organic products.

If you stick to the natural foods which Mother Nature provides, your body will work in balancing itself and maintaining a suitable weight. Know that organic foods come without toxic chemicals (a typical apple comes with 20 - 30 artificial toxins on its skin). Research has shown that organic foods come with around 50% more minerals, vitamins, enzymes, as well as other micronutrients in comparison to non-organic foods. Organic foods are known to last longer, taste better, and since your body will get its share of nutrients in smaller portions, you will also be eating less.

Q & A

Is organic food better for my health?

Yes. Since the use of pesticides and chemical fertilizers is absent from organic foods, and since this minimizes our exposure to toxic elements, organic foods automatically become healthier alternatives in comparison to conventionally grown/manufactured food. In addition various studies have shown health benefits of organic foods vs their non-organic counterparts.

A research carried out in Europe by the Danish Institute of Agricultural Research, the Institute of Grassland and Environmental Research, and the University of Aberdeen, showed that organic milk produced by pasture grazed cows had more vitamins, CLA, antioxidants, and omega 3, in comparison to commercially farmed milk.

A study carried out at the University of California which spanned a ten year period showed that organically grown tomatoes came with a significantly higher percentage of antioxidants.

A UK based paper published in 2004 stated that eating an organic diet helps minimize the ingestion of toxic chemicals; reduces your expose to food additives and colours; helps you avoid genetically modified foods; increases your intake of micronutrients like antioxidants, minerals, & vitamins, and can also work in lowering the risk of contracting conditions like coronary heart disease and cancers.

Is organic meat/dairy/eggs better for the farm animals?

Yes. It is common knowledge that normal living conditions in most commercial feedlots and farms prevent animals from growing and developing normally.

For instance, commercially farmed hens often live in cages which are too small for them to even turn around, and are bred at much faster rates in comparison to a few decades ago. Death due to heart & lung complications in such situations is not uncommon, and compromised immune systems lead to the use of antibiotics. Commercially raised cattle are typically fed high grain diets (cows are NOT designed to eat grains, they are only designed to eat grass. When fed grains, the cow becomes fatter, as fat cells store toxins.) which can lead to high acid build up and even death.

The production of organic foods ensures that animals are not confined in small spaces, where the chickens are free range and the cattle are grass fed. Livestock is typically fed organically grown feed, and when it comes to health, the use of antibiotics is all but absent.

Organic practises ensure that livestock is provided with stress free and comfortable living conditions based on the needs of the species in question. Common practises include ensuring round-the-clock access to open air, suitable forage/pasture, limiting transportation, prohibiting isolating or permanent tethering of animals, and providing suitable bedding.

In addition, mutilation in the form of removal or reduction of tails, beaks, and horns, is also prohibited.

How do I know if something is organic?

The simplest way to find out if something is organic is to refer to the label. However, labelling of organic food can vary from nation to nation.

For instance, the USDA has created three different categories when it comes to the labelling of organic products wherein products made using 100% organic products can be labelled '100% organic'; products which contain at least 95% organic ingredients can be labelled 'organic'; and products made using at least 70% organic ingredients can be labelled 'made with organic ingredients'.

The Canadian Food Inspection Agency allows producers/ manufacturers to use 'Biologique Canada' or 'Canada Organic' if the product in question is made using at least 95% organic ingredients. In case a product comes with 70 – 95% organic ingredients, the labelling should tell you the exact percentage.

Why does organic food cost more?

Organic foods can cost between 10 – 40% more than their conventional counterparts. Producing organic food is more expensive in comparison to producing non-organic food. Not being able to use pesticides, for instance, results in increased manual costs because in such a scenario hand-weeding would be required.

The fact that organic farming is often carried out on small scales also adds to their being more expensive. Animal feed, which is mainly organic, is more expensive than regular feed as well.

What are the benefits of eating organic?

Organic fruits and vegetables, as mentioned, are grown without the use of chemical fertilizers, herbicides, and pesticides; and when it comes to animal based food products, there is no use of antibiotics or hormones. The most visible benefit of eating organic, therefore, is that you limit the amount of harmful toxins and preservatives finding their way into your system.

A research carried out at the University of California showed that organically grown corn and berries had more than 50% polyphenolics (antioxidants) and considerably more ascorbic acid in comparison to produce grown conventionally in a neighbouring plot. A study carried out at the University of Washington showed that children who were on organic diets had six times lower pesticide levels in their bodies in comparison to children who consumed conventionally grown and produced foods.

Apart from health benefits, organic farming also helps protect the soil and is believed to result in yields that are three times higher when compared to conventional farming. Since most organic foods are grown and produced locally, being on an organic diet also helps support the local economy.

Why choose organic vegetables? Are frozen veggies just as good as fresh ... why or why not?

You'll find that you will eat LESS certified organic foods; as smaller portions contain the same, if not more nutrients than portions twice the size that are not organic.

Nothing is as good as fresh. That being said, a lot of the 'fresh' veggies in the store have actually been picked weeks or even months before. Some have been irradiated to delay ripening (and kill bacteria). These 'fresh' veggies will not have the same nutrient value as a vegetable locally grown and picked recently.

If a vegetable is not in season and you can't get it fresh, I'll suggest frozen as a second best option. Typically frozen veggies are picked when ripe, and frozen right away. This will allow you to have vegetables even when they are not in season. I'll even suggest this option, as it is convenient and most don't eat enough vegetables in a day to maintain good health. I'll suggest eating 3-8 cups of non starchy vegetables a day.

What are some of the basic "rules' when it comes to eating naturally.

Simple...If it comes from Mother Nature and is not processed, it is natural. If it comes from man and is processed, it's not natural. For example, we are often told that bread and pasta made from whole grain sources are good for us. Last time I checked, there was no pasta bush, or bread tree. That means bread and pasta don't come from Mother Nature. These are man made, processed foods. Man has taken a whole food made in nature and processed it, so the food is no longer natural. It is very, very convenient; but no longer natural. Basic rule of thumb: If it grows, eat it.

There are a lot of food products that say they are natural ... how can someone tell how natural they are?

This is a loaded question as the current labelling laws allow for A LOT of misleading information to be on our food labels. The only way to know your foods are indeed natural would be to buy your meat and produce from a local farmer. Meet the farmer. Ask questions. Go to the farm and see how your food is being grown or raised. Shop at your local farmers market. If you must shop in a grocery store, look for Certified Organic Labels. Avoid canned, boxed, and pre-packaged foods whenever possible.

Why is it important to know how my food is raised, processed and brought to me in the grocery store?

You ARE what you eat. It is essential that you know what you are eating. Not many of us pay enough attention to what we eat and drink, and most of these will come as a surprise to you.

- Did you know your 100% pure juice in a carton is pasteurized?
- Even organic milk sold in stores is pasteurized.
- Did you know the baby carrots in a bag are dipped in chlorine to keep them looking fresh and orange in color? (notice how they turn white when left out)
- Fruits and vegetables - even organically grown varieties - may have cow-, pig-, and chicken collagen coatings on them, or wax, as well as a number of other unsavoury ingredients. (MAP - modified Atmosphere packaging)
- Commercially farmed animals are fed sawdust, drywall dust,

and grains to fatten up before slaughter; and fed antibiotics and growth hormones as well.
- Be aware of meat glue.
- Be aware of chemical additives for 'flavour'.

What is Pasteurization?

Pasteurization involves heating the product in order to kill any harmful bacteria. The problem is that the heating process kills the healthy enzymes and bacteria, and damages or destroys the vitamins and amino acids as well.

Pasteurized foods therefore are not healthy choices. These foods that were once a healthy choice, have been processed into an unhealthy choice. Avoid pasteurized foods whenever possible.

What is the truth about microwaving?

Here are facts you should know.

- Small amounts of radiation leaks through the glass of the microwave.
- Microwaving damages the cell wall of your food and your body no longer recognizes it as food, which may lead to an immune response.
- Heating food in a microwave destroys nutrients and antioxidants originally in the food making it less nutritious
- It really is GREAT for disinfecting your kitchen sponges if put in wet.

What are the pros and cons of using a microwave?

Pros
- Putting a WET kitchen sponge or cloth in a microwave for 2 minutes, will kill up to 99% of harmful bacteria

Cons

- Foods lose nutrients when cooked in a microwave
- Chemical structure of food changes when cooked in a microwave
- Toxins leach from plastic used to heat food in a microwave

A study published in the November 2003 issue of The Journal of the Science of Food and Agriculture found that broccoli "zapped" in the microwave with a little water lost up to 97 percent of the beneficial antioxidant chemicals it contains. By comparison, steamed broccoli lost 11 percent or fewer of its antioxidants.

What are your personal top 5 healthy foods?

In no particular order of preference, these have got to be it.

- Raw Chocolate (see **www.sacredchocolate.com**) – great antioxidant and tastes fantastic
- Extra Virgin Certified Organic Coconut Oil – healthiest fat on earth
- Certified Organic Fruits (berries are best) – filled with vitamins, minerals and antioxidants
- Certified Organic Veggies (green leafy veggies like Kale are best) – Filled with vitamins and minerals
- Certified Organic Meat (Beef, Poultry, Eggs, Wild Fish, Wild Game) – high in healthy proteins, fats, vitamins and minerals

NOTES:

NUTRITION - THE BASICS

Q & A

What are the benefits of healthy eating?

Eating healthy essentially means eating foods in their natural form and steering clear of all kinds of processed foods.

It is scientifically proven in many studies, that what you eat has a significant bearing on how you feel. The benefits of eating healthy are diverse, and here are the most important ones.

Keeping your health in check:

One of the best reasons to get on a healthy eating plan is to help prevent and keep in check a large number of medical conditions: high blood pressure, heart disease, type-2 diabetes, as well as certain kinds of cancer. There is an abundance on research linking diseases to unhealthy eating patterns.

Preventing obesity and tackling weight loss:

Healthy eating patterns help prevent obesity, and the same can also be said when it comes to tackling weight loss. The great thing about eating healthy in order to lose weight, is that you do not have to starve yourself; you simply have to eat right for you.

Better mental health:

Various studies show that people with healthy eating habits are normally happier in comparison with people who do not have healthy eating habits. This is because healthy food supplies the body with the nutrients it needs to repair, rebuild and even helps increase the brain's serotonin levels (the happy hormone).

Providing energy:

If you eat right, you will find no need for caffeine in coffee, tea, energy drinks or energy bars to get you going. A healthy diet for you will ensure that you get all your required energy on an everyday basis.

Providing skin and hair care:

Eating healthy for you will ensure that your body is exposed to limited toxins. Toxins can cause pimples, eczema, psoriasis, brittle, dull and dry hair. By eating healthy, your skin and hair will feel the positive difference.

What are the consequences of a poor diet?

A simple example of an unhealthy diet is one that depends on convenience; fast foods, fried foods, chips, pizzas, and all but eliminating fresh fruits and vegetables. Eating unhealthy could also mean eating at odd times by not giving your body the time it needs to digest what you've eaten, or by spacing your meals too far apart.

Deficiency:

A poor diet is a certain path for the body to miss out on getting vital nutrients; this can lead to various problems . For instance, vitamin A deficiency can cause night blindness; vitamin K deficiency can cause haemorrhages (bleeding). One study even linked deficiency in zinc to aggressive behaviour, wherein the subjects showed signs of decreased aggression upon being treated with zinc in therapeutic doses.

Weight worries:

The SAD diet (Standard American Diet) clearly isn't working for us as a nation. The suggestion to eat 'higher fibre, lower fat' diets have not led us to improved health; this eating plan instead has led to 67% of society being considered overweight. Eating convenience foods instead of eating healthy foods has most people seeking a miracle diet to help them find and maintain a healthy weight. The miracle diet is simple... Eat the way mother nature intended. When you choose convenience instead, you welcome an unhealthy weight and the worries that go with it.

Mind matters:

While a healthy diet promotes mental health, an unhealthy diet can lead to irritability, mood swings, disturbed sleep, giddiness, lack of concentration, and in cases, even depression. Multiple studies have shown that an improved diet improves mental health.

What are the basic food groups?

Foods, based on their nutritional properties, are divided into basic food groups, and each plays an important role in our overall nutrition. The basic food groups include the following.

- **Whole Grains**: rice, buckwheat, oats, quinoa, wheat
- **Fruits**: Apples, berries, peaches, plums, pears
- **Vegetables**: Lettuce, broccoli, cabbage, okra, potatoes, carrots
- **Raw** Dairy: Butter, cheese, milk, yogurt
- **Meat**: Chicken, beef, fish, pork, wild game
- **Nuts/seeds/legumes**: Almonds, beans, cashew nuts, lentils, peas, etc.
- **Oils/fats**: Vegetable oils, coconut oil, animal fat

Why do you think CFG (Canada's Food Guide) is killing us as a nation?

- I do not support Canada's Food Guide. I believe it is inadequate as guideline for health.
- Too many carbohydrate foods are suggested. We DO NOT need grains as outlined. Too many carbohydrates lead to increased fat, insulin resistance, and are a huge contributor to our obesity epidemic today.
- Condones processed, packaged, refined foods – toxic to our health.
- Suggests decreasing fats from natural sources. We NEED healthy fats to be healthy.
- Not enough healthy fats are suggested.
- No separations are made between fruits and veggies (fruit should be limited and GREEN leafy veggies increased).
- 98% of the population are sensitive to dairy, and it is an entire food group. ELIMINATE DAIRY!
- Meat and alternatives are too low. Diet could be 10-40% required for protein.
- No explanations are given for age groups, or activity level, or ethnicity, or current weight.

Why is it important to vary your food choices?

Eating the same foods can lead to food sensitivity, intolerance and even allergy. Rotating your food promotes variety in your diet, improves digestion and helps your body detoxify. The easiest way to avoid this is to rotate your foods every 4 days. For example, if you have oatmeal on Monday, don't have Oatmeal again until Friday. I suggest you start your rotation day at dinner. That way you can take your dinner leftovers for lunch the next day. So beef one day, pork the next, fish the next, and chicken the next, for example. Consider a food rotation diet every few months to allow your digestive system to improve.

NOTES:

Understanding Nutrients

What are nutrients?

Nutrients, simply put, are chemicals that your body needs in order to carry on with its day-to-day functioning. Different nutrients play different roles, some of which include regulating bodily functions, building & repairing tissue and providing energy, to name a few.

Nutrients are classified under two basic categories; macronutrients, and micronutrients.

Macronutrients: are ones which are required in significantly large volumes.

Micronutrients: are ones which are required in smaller volumes.

Carbohydrates, protein, fats, and water fall under macronutrients. Vitamins and minerals constitute as micronutrients.

A healthy diet should ideally incorporate all of these in the right quantities, although quantities of each will vary from person to person. For your specific ratios, I'll suggest 'Metabolic Typing' by William Wolcott.

The six main nutrients are:

- Carbohydrates
- Fats
- Minerals
- Protein
- Vitamins
- Water

MACRONUTRIENTS:

Carbohydrates

O f all the nutrients our bodies need, none has received more attention than carbohydrates. Should your diet be high carb, low carb, no carb.... The controversy, and the misinformation, has reached epic proportion. To try to break through all of the myths, here are a few facts about carbohydrates.

Carbohydrates are your body's main fuel source. Your body's every function is dependent on carbohydrate fuel. Breathing, walking, thinking, talking... All of these actions require energy. Without proper fuel, your body will not function at its best. Your body requires at least 40-60% of its daily calories from carbohydrate sources.

Carbohydrates are found in all foods, (with the exception of meat and eggs) primarily in grains, fruits, vegetables, and milk products. (RAW is best as Pasteurized has less nutrient value). Not all carbohydrates are created equal! High quality carbohydrates come from brown rice, whole grains such as quinoa or amaranth and fruits and vegetables. These provide the fiber, vitamins and minerals to keep your body functioning at its best. Low quality carbohydrates, such as breads, pasta, white rice and donuts, cookies, candy and sugar, will not provide as much nutritional value and are often high in calories and harmful, unhealthy fat.

Carbohydrates are broken down and provide a source of energy in about 20 minutes, lasting up to 4 hours (depending on the carbohydrate). The longer it takes food to digest, the longer you feel full. This is called satiety. Foods with a higher fiber content have a higher satiety level, as do foods with protein and/or fats in them. To get the most out of your carbohydrates, try to combine them with a protein/fat at each meal. You can do this by pairing a grain, vegetable or fruit with a meat, raw milk product or fat. See the chart on page 38 for a few carb/protein/fat ideas.

So why are low carb/ high protein diets so popular these days? The unfortunate truth is that these diets do work in the short term - you will lose weight on them. The question is, what kind of weight will you lose, and at what cost?

To understand why these diets don't work and why eating carbohydrates is so important, here are a few energy basics.

When you eat carbohydrates, they are broken down into glycogen. Glycogen is energy that is very easily broken down and used by your body. Glycogen is transported through your bloodstream to the part of your body that needs fuel. If your body doesn't currently need energy, the glycogen is transported to your organs. If your organs don't need that energy, the glycogen is converted into stored energy - body fat.

When your body requires energy, first it looks to the bloodstream. If there is no glycogen available, your body will look to the organs. If there is no glycogen available there, then your body will turn to stored energy to convert for fuel. This is the premise that low carb/ high protein diets are based on.

In actuality, when there are no carbohydrates present, it is very difficult for your body to break down fat and convert it into energy. When your body converts fat into fuel without the presence of glycogen, ketone bodies are produced. Ketone bodies are noted for their appetite-suppressing effect, but also cause dehydration by increased urination, weakness, dizziness, bad breath and headaches. If your body is in ketosis for long enough, you are at risk for gout, renal disease and kidney stones because of increased uric acid levels. (Ketoacidosis can be FATAL for diabetics)

Without sufficient carbohydrates, your body will also use protein stores for fuel. Unfortunately, your body does not have the capability to store protein; so the stores it turns to is your muscle tissue. A low carb diet will result in significant loss of lean muscle tissue, which results in a decrease in your metabolism and weight gain will follow.

Other results of high-protein, low-carb diets include osteoporosis (due to an increased loss of calcium in the urine), fainting spells (due to loss of fluid and electrolytes) and an inability to think effectively (as your brain can not store its own fuel, it relies on your body providing adequate fuel).

The answer to the question "high or low carb?" is BALANCE. Each food contains nutrients that are essential for proper health – and a body that is not healthy will have a harder time achieving a healthy weight. It's important to eat a VARIETY of foods in MODERATION.

Another reason that any healthy eating plan must contain carbohydrates is that they contain fiber. Fiber is found only in plant foods- vegetables, fruits, whole grains, and are important for three main reasons:

1. Fiber slows down the passage of food through the intestines. This is important because the vitamins and minerals that we need are absorbed here. Eating enough fiber ensures the proper absorption of the nutrients that our body needs.

2. The longer it takes food to digest, the longer you feel full! Foods with a high fiber content will keep you feeling fuller for longer - which means that you won't have to eat as much to feel satisfied.

3.Everyone knows this one - fiber keeps you regular! This is vital because eliminating regularly rids your body of the toxins and wastes that can be harmful to your body. It's also been proven that a diet rich in fiber helps to prevent colon and other cancers. Having 1 to 3 bowel movements every day is a sign of good health. Ideally, your poop should be:

- Approximately 12 inches per day (1 -12 inch, 2-6 inch or 3-4inch poops per day)
- Easy to pass
- Earthy in smell
- Formed, but not hard
- No food particles seen

On the other hand:

- If you are experiencing diarrhea, your body may be trying to detoxify. Reduce refined and processed foods, and choose whole, natural foods to help detoxify.
- If you are experiencing pellet poops, you may be dehydrated. Drink more water.
- If you are experiencing large, hard to pass (feels square) poops, you may be consuming too many processed foods. Reduce the processed foods and choose whole, natural foods.
- If you are experiencing poop that floats but won't flush the first time, you may not be producing enough bile to break down fats. See a Naturopath or Natural Nutritionist to give you a liver cleansing diet.
- If you are experiencing food particles in your poop, you may not be chewing your foods enough. Try chewing your foods until liquefied.
- If you are experiencing really stinky poops, it's time to detoxify! See a Naturopath or Natural Nutritionist to give you a detox diet.

There are two types of fiber. Soluble fiber can be dissolved in water, helps to lower blood cholesterol levels and helps to control blood sugar levels in people with diabetes. Soluble fiber can be found in apples, plums, oranges, brussel sprouts, carrots, legumes, barley, oatbran, and psyllium. Insoluble fiber absorbs water, giving bulk to your stool and preventing constipation and hemorrhoids. Organic Whole grains, brown rice, corn, fruits with edible seeds and the skins of most fruits and vegetables are excellent sources of insoluble fiber.

Getting enough fiber - 25 to 40 grams each day - isn't as hard as you think. Legumes, such as split peas, lentils and chick peas have 5 to 7 grams in half a cup, while 1 cup of beans has approximately 15 grams.

Eating 25 to 40 grams of fiber per day can also:

- Prevent heart disease
- Lower cholesterol
- Lower risk of blood clots
- Prevents constipation and hemorrhoids
- Prevents colon and other cancers
- Lessen insulin required by people with Type 1 Diabetes

By eating 5 to 10 servings of vegetables and fruits and whole grains every day throughout the course of the day, you'll get the fiber you need from your diet. Get the most fiber out of your vegetables and fruits by eating them with the skin on.

Great snack ideas: Goal – combine carbohydrate with a protein or fat.

Whole Grain, Vegetable or Fruit	Eat with Raw Milk Product, Meat or Beans/legumes
Quinoa or rice	Black Beans
Berries, apples, pears etc	Raw Yogurt or cottage cheese
Whole Grain granola	Raw Yogurt
Salad	Tuna or chick peas, nuts or seeds, Raw cottage cheese
Sprouted Grain Pita	Hummus
1/3 cup dried fruit	¼ cup nuts
Raw veggies	Dip or salad dressing (make yourself)

Q & A

What happens if I eat too many carbohydrates - what does my body do with it?

The body ends up storing carbohydrates as fats, and this reserve is used in the event that the body does not get enough energy through carbohydrates. Eating too much in the form of carbohydrates can cause weight gain/obesity, especially if the diet comprises mainly of refined processed carbohydrates (bread, pasta, cakes, crackers, bagels etc.)

What are some good sources of Carbohydrates?

Good sources of carbohydrates include whole grains, fruits, vegetables, and beans. Steer clear of refined carbohydrates that come in the form of refined grains as well as any kind of processed carbohydrate based food. Breads, cereals, pasta, cakes, crackers, bagels etc.

My best Carbohydrate choices:
Grains
- Quiona
- Rice
- Oats
- Millet
- Buckwheat
- Amaranth
- Arrowroot
- Corn (certified organic only)

Fruits
- Apples
- Peaches
- Pears
- Plums
- All berries
- Tropical Fruits
- Cherries
- Watermelon
- Tomato
- Citrus Fruits
- Lemon/Lime
- Dates/Figs
- Grapes
- Avocado
- Apricot

Vegetables
- Salad made with:
  - Spinach
  - Kale
  - Iceberg
  - Butter

- Romaine
- Mesclun Mix
- Chard
- Collard Green
- Dandelion Greens

- Onions
- Mushrooms
- Garlic
- Asparagus
- Celery
- Cucumber
- Beets
- Broccoli
- Brussel Sprouts
- Cabbage
- Carrots
- Cauliflower
- Eggplant
- Peas
- Red, Green, Yellow, Orange Peppers
- Parsnip
- Pumpkin
- All Sea Vegetables
- Alfalfa
- Sprouts
- Chinese Vegetables
- Beans
- Potatoes
- Yams
- Sweet Potatoes

What's the problem with gluten?

According to the CHEK Institute, about 2/3 of us are gluten sensitive. Approximately 1 out of every 133 are Celiac. Visit www.celiac.ca for more information.

Gluten, along with Dairy are among this country's top allergen foods. The others are corn, shellfish, soy, chocolate (sorry to be the bearer of horrible news on that one), eggs and citrus fruits.

I've never met anyone who was gluten intolerant and not dairy intolerant too. So here's a good reason to eliminate the gluten and the dairy at the same time.

Gluten comes from the Latin word meaning Glue. This is what holds breads together. This is the glue that will interfere with the breakdown and absorption of nutrients, leading to constipation. This clump of glue can't be digested; this triggers your immune system to attack the lining of your small intestine. This leads to pain, bloating, diarrhoea or constipation.

Keep eating Gluten, ignoring the negative symptoms you are experiencing, and your small intestine can become damaged, and less and less able to absorb nutrients from all the foods you eat. This leads to malnutrition, even though you are eating more and more.

Eating gluten can lead to osteoporosis, nervous system diseases, anaemia, weight loss, weight gain, depression, fatigue, early menopause or even infertility.

Look for foods that are labelled 'Gluten Free'. Even foods that don't contain gluten can be contaminated with gluten due to the processing. It's a pretty safe bet to say if it comes in a can, a box or is made by man; it will have some form of gluten.

The list of gluten free foods is HUGE. Visit www.celiac.ca for more information.

Should I choose whole grains over a flour source?

Whole grains come from Nature and flour comes from Man processing those whole grains. This process of making flour denatures the food, which means you won't get the same nutritional benefit from flour. Flour is hard for your body to process as it is a gluey substance, and can interfere with the breakdown of food and absorption of nutrients. Choose Whole Grains. Great whole grains include quinoa, rice, amaranth, corn, buckwheat, millet, and oats. These are all great for those who are gluten intolerant. For those who are not, you can choose whole grains including barley, wheat, rye and kamut to name a few.

How much Carbohydrates should the average person have a day and a meal?

- Start with 50% of your daily caloric intake (See page 60 to Calculate your caloric needs) from carbohydrates, 25% from fat and 25% from protein.
- If you are very active, you may need up to 70% of each meal from carbohydrates. If you are inactive, you may need as little as 30% of each meal from carbohydrate.
- To learn about your individual needs, I'll suggest you meet with a Natural Nutritionist or Naturopathic Doctor to make a specific meal plan for you.
- You will also learn from the book, 'Metabolic Typing' by William Wolcott.

Protein

Protein is essential for your body to grow and develop healthfully. It makes up the second largest component of your body, water being the first. It also provides structure for hormones, antibodies, enzymes, muscle, ligaments, hair, skin, nails and tissues. Protein is a very important nutrient when you are under a great deal of stress.

According to the Canadian Association of Fitness Professionals, the human stress response can increase caloric need by up to 200%, and the need for protein by 60-500%! Your body requires at least 15-30% of its daily calories from Protein.

Protein is broken down into amino acids – referred to as the "building blocks" of protein. Your body can produce several of these; they are called non-essential amino acids. The human body cannot produce 9 of these so they must be procured from food. These are called Essential amino acids.

When your body makes protein- (for example when it's repairing muscle tissue), it needs a variety of amino acids. If one or more amino acids are not present (either from your body, or from your food), your body is unable to produce the protein necessary for the repair.

Protein is found in all foods, and is categorized in two groups. A complete protein contains ample amounts of all essential amino acids, and can be found in animal sources such as meat, fish, raw dairy, raw cheese, eggs and raw milk. Incomplete proteins are generally found in plant foods such as nuts, seeds, grains, legumes (beans, split peas, lentils, chick peas) and have one or more essential amino acids missing.

This does not mean, however, that all of your protein must come from animal sources. Because plant proteins are not complete, they need to be combined with another incomplete protein to supply your body with all necessary essential amino acids. Use the following chart to create complete proteins by combining foods.

Add variety to your eating plan by putting nuts or seeds on your salads. (1/4 cup is one serving). Legumes (chick peas, lentils and beans) are high in fiber, inexpensive and a good source of protein.

Like many nutrients, eating too much protein can be just as harmful as not eating enough. Unlike fat and carbohydrates, your body cannot store protein. A diet too high in protein can put strain on the liver and kidneys and may cause kidney stones.

Not sure about Plant Proteins? Try these:
- Chili made with a variety of legumes and vegetables
- Mushroom burgers
- Hummus – a Mediterranean spread made with chick peas, served with whole wheat pitas
- On salad – nuts, seeds, chickpeas or mixed beans
- Mixed bean salad
- Split pea or bean soup
- Add lentils to a stir-fry instead of meat

Protein Combining Chart

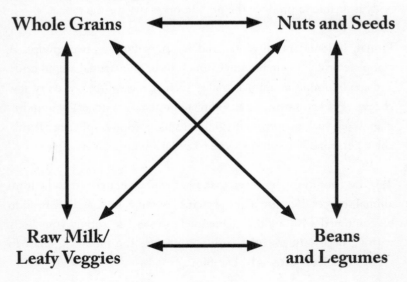

Q & A

What happens if I eat too much Protein - what does my body do with it?

Too much protein may lead to toxins building up in the body (called Ketones), and the kidneys will then flush these toxins, which can lead to kidney and liver stress, dehydration and mineral loss.

What happens if I do not eat enough Protein?

If you are working hard to build your body and not eating enough protein, your workout efforts will be futile. And without enough protein your nails won't grow, you'll have dull or breaking hair, and it's likely you'll suffer from headaches or migraines.

What are some good sources of Protein?

Choose certified organic, free range sources.

- Beef
- Wild Game
- Wild Fish/Shellfish
- Eggs
- Pork
- Chicken
- Turkey

See the above chart for non meat sources of protein.

How much Protein should the average person have a day and a meal?

- Start with 25% of your daily caloric intake coming from protein, (See page 60 to Calculate your caloric needs). 25% from fat and 50% from Carbohydrates.
- Adjust your ratios based on your activity level, stress level, current state of health, metabolism and muscle mass.

To learn about your individual needs, I'll suggest you meet with a Natural Nutritionist or Naturopathic Doctor to make a specific meal plan for you.

You will also learn from the book, 'Metabolic Typing' by William Wolcott.

Can I take in all the protein I need from supplements? Why and why not?

No. Nature's foods provide all the nutrients and enzymes we need to utilize the foods and improve our health. This cannot be said for all supplements. Remember, supplements are processed and often manufactured from man made sources. No supplement will ever provide you with the same quality and nutrient value as food from nature.

As our lives can sometimes be hectic, a protein supplement may be used, although I don't believe protein supplements should be used as a staple in any diet.

Whey protein is by far the most commonly used protein supplement, and is amongst the two kinds one can find in milk (casein being the other). Whey is derived as a by-product during the making of cheese, wherein while the casein remains in the cheese, whey becomes part of the watery residue.

In choosing whey protein based products you have several options; these include whey protein concentrates and isolates. People who suffer from lactose intolerance or sensitivity to dairy products are best off relying on whey protein isolate as it comes with negligible quantities of lactose and fat, and a very high percentage of protein concentration.

What would you suggest as high protein snacks on the go?

Boiled eggs, nuts/seeds, pre cooked chicken/beef/pork slices, beans/legumes, and raw organic cheese.

Is soy a good protein source?

Soy is not a healthy choice. This is simply because almost all soy is now Genetically Modified and contains goitrogens which suppresses thyroid function. In addition:

- Soy is high in phytic acid causing decrease in absorption of minerals.
- Soybeans contain haemagglutinin, a clot-promoting substance that causes red blood cells to clump together which leads to cancer.
- Soy blocks calcium and leads to vitamin D deficiencies.
- 100 grams of soy protein has the estrogenic equivalent of the pill (100gr soy contains a toxic level of almost 600mg of isoflavones).

What is meat glue and is it any good?

The use of Meat glue scares me.

Meat processing plants use an enzyme called transglutaminase (approved for use in USA and Canada) to glue bits of meat and meat trim together to make steaks, and apparently, even butchers can't taste or tell the difference.

The process of making it involves taking scraps/pieces of meat that would normally be thrown out and gluing them together to look like a whole piece of meat, and it is being sold in stores as real steak.

Potential health hazards - bits are exposed to air and bacteria, then put together allowing for a breeding ground inside the reconstituted steaks. They must then be cooked thoroughly and not be served rare or medium.

In Canada 'transglutaminase' must appear on label if used to process any product.

Is Dairy a good protein source?

Pasteurized Dairy is not a healthy choice. Raw Dairy is a healthy choice.

If all you have access to is pasteurized milk, cheese or butter, then I'll suggest you skip it altogether. Remember, Pasteurization destroys vitamins and amino acids, rendering dairy a poor protein source.

Is milk from almond, rice or soy a better choice?

Yes. They are better choices than the milk you can buy in the grocery store, although in Canada almond milk and rice milk as they are sold in the store are pasteurized and lack the nutrients we think we are getting. Soy in any form is not a food I'd recommend due to Genetic Modification and the Estrogenic Effects.

Fat

Contrary to what you might think, fat is a necessary nutrient in your healthy eating plan. Fat is essential for health, and has many functions to keep your body working at its best. Fat provides concentrated energy for our bodies to use when there is no other available energy, fat insulates and protects our organs, it carries fat soluble vitamins A, D, E and K and regulates body temperature.

There are several components of fat, some of which are harmful and should be limited, and some which are essential and must be a part of your diet. In order to understand which is which, you much first understand the components of fat.

Cholesterol is found in all animal fats and oils, and is also produced in the body by your liver. Cholesterol is essential for maintaining nerve and brain tissue, producing bile for digestion, and forming vitamin D and several hormones. Generally, your liver will produce as much cholesterol as your body needs. Any cholesterol that you take in through your diet is stored for future use. Cholesterol is carried through your bloodstream by two kinds of LipoProteins.

Low Density LipoProteins (LDL's) carry cholesterol to your organs and cells, and along the way deposit it in your arteries. Over time, this will lead to blockages in the arteries, which in turn can lead to a heart attack. High Density LipoProteins (HDL's) on the other hand, transport cholesterol from the blood and tissues, ridding the body of the artery-clogging fatty deposits. Exercise has a very positive effect on HDL levels, while smoking increases LDL levels.

Cholesterol that you eat in food,(egg yolks for example), has very little to do with the cholesterol level in your blood. Genetics, your activity level, and the amount of Trans fat (man made foods, fast food, margarine, or packaged foods) in your diet have the most impact.

Saturated fats are primarily found in animal sources, and are solid at room temperature (for example, bacon fat and lard). The BEST fat you can consume comes from Certified Oganic, Extra Virgin Coconut oil. This can be used at high temperature cooking. (and can also be used as an incredible skin moisturizer!)

There are two types of unsaturated fat: Polyunsaturated fats are found in corn, safflower and sunflower oils and increases HDL's, lowering your cholesterol level. Monounsaturated fats are found in vegetable, nut, canola and olive oil. This fat lowers LDL levels in the blood, lowering your cholesterol level.

Essential fatty acids (EFA's, collectively known as vitamin F) are found in every healthy cell in the body, and are important for normal growth in cells, muscles, nerves and organs. EFA's are also used to produce certain hormones. Deficiencies of EFA's are linked to a variety of health problems, including heart disease, cancer and diabetes. EFA's are classified in two types: Omega-3 and Omega-6 fatty acids.

Omega-3 appears to reduce cardiovascular disease by raising HDL levels and is found in:
- cold-water fish (salmon, tuna, sardines, halibut, herring, mackerel and trout)
- walnuts
- flax
- green leafy vegetables

Omega-6 is found more easily in the average North American diet and is found in:
- Nuts and seeds
- Safflower oil
- Olive oil
- Sunflower oil
- Corn oil
- Evening Primrose oil
- Borage oils

Proper balance between omega-3 and omega-6 is important, a ratio of 1 to 1 is recommended. Because omega-6 is so readily available, that increases the need for omega-3s. Cut back on Omega- 6 and increase Omega-3 to help balance your body.

Trans-Fatty Acids are Man-made and produced when liquid fats are hydrogenated or turned into solid fats (for example, margarine and shortening). Trans-Fatty Acids can disrupt the processing of EFA's. Your body has only one enzyme to break down fatty acids. If you consume Trans-Fatty acids, the enzyme breaks down those first, leaving the healthy essential fatty acids unprocessed. For this reason, be very careful of consuming trans-fats. Many low fat prepared foods such as cookies and crackers can be very high is trans-fats. Read labels carefully to ensure your food choices do not contain them.

The amount of fat in your diet is important on many levels. An unbalanced diet leads to heart disease and certain cancers. But because fat makes food taste good, digests slowly (keeping you feeling fuller for longer), and is essential for health, you do not want to restrict fat from your diet. We recommend a diet of approximately 30% fat from Natural sources.

Q & A

What happens if I eat too much fat?

If you are a regular eater of unhealthy trans fats (fast food, packaged, canned, processed, restaurant), you can experience weight gain due to toxicity; and you could also become prone to contracting heart and liver diseases.

Eating healthy fats (nuts, seeds, fish, meats, eggs, avocado, coconut oil) will not make you fat anymore than eating money will make you rich.

What happens if I do not eat enough Fat?

You can expect hormone imbalance, brain fog, constipation, joint discomfort and poor energy to name a few. Your neural pathways are insulated with fat, and the absence of fat can lead to depression, PMS and serious and irreversible nerve problems.

What are some good sources of Fat?

Coconut oil, fish, flax, chia seeds, hemp, wild game, Free Range grass fed animals, vegetables like avocadoes and olives; nuts like almonds, cashews, walnuts, and hazelnuts; nut butter and butter are all some good sources of good fats.

You should avoid man made foods that include Trans Fats, cakes, pastries, crackers, candy bars, and cookies and all things deep fried.

How much Fat should the average person have a day and a meal?

- Start with 25% of your daily caloric intake coming from fats (See page 60 to Calculate your caloric needs), 25 % from Protein and 50% from carbohydrates.
- You can increase or decrease this percentage based on how you feel. For example, when you eat, you should not feel hungry for 2-4 hours.
- If you are hungry sooner than that, I'll suggest you increase your fats as they help you feel satiated for longer.
- To learn about your individual needs, I'll suggest you meet with a Natural Nutritionist or Naturopathic Doctor to make a specific meal plan for you.
- You will also learn from the book, 'Metabolic Typing' by William Wolcott.

What is the difference between butter and margarine?

Butter is filled with nutrients like Vitamin A, D, E, K, selenium and fatty acids that all come from a natural source and improve our body's health.

Margarine is man made and is filled with synthetic vitamins, trans fats, preservatives, colors and artificial flavours and is more of a food like substance than a real food.

Butter is healthy for your body. Margarine of all kinds is toxic to your body. Choose butter for better heart health, digestion and the growth and development of your healthy body.

What are the best fats to cook with?

Choosing healthy cooking oils requires particular attention, because oils tend to produce unhealthy chemicals when exposed to heat. In fact, while monounsaturated fats are otherwise considered a healthy form of fat; they also become unhealthy upon heating.

The best oils for you to use when frying are Coconut oil or Ghee, as these oils remain stable at high heat.

NO HEAT oils include Fish, Flax, Borage, Hemp seed, and Cod Liver oil

Oils to use while baking include Pumpkin and sunflower oil.

Oils to use for light sautéing include Olive, Sesame, Pistachio and Grape Seed oil

Water

Water plays a crucial role in our diets, and some of its most important functions include:
- Transporting oxygen/nutrients through blood
- Aiding in the digestive process
- Regulating temperature
- Providing cells shape & stability

- Enabling a host of chemical reactions to take place within the body

Research has shown that water can also play an important role when it comes to tackling weight loss; this is because it provides the body with hydration, without any calories. Drinking water before meals can give you a fuller feeling allowing you to eat less. In addition, drinking water also helps the body flush out waste- this is particularly important in any weight loss goal.

Q & A

How much should we drink and why?

How much water should you actually be drinking? In truth, I have no idea. It totally depends. My general rule of thumb is simple. When you pee, it should be clear or the color of lemonade. For some to reach that point, it may be 8 cups or less. For others it may be 12 or more. Some factors that determine the amount of water you need include; your activity level, how much you sweat, how dry the climate is where you live, the foods you eat, the altitude of where you live, how much caffeine you drink and even how much you speak in a day.

Start with 8 cups of water per day and add more if you ever feel thirsty or your pee is still yellow.

What "type" should we drink?

When I say drink water, I DO NOT mean tap water. Tap water is toxic. Depending on where you live, your tap water may contain fluoride, chlorine, aluminum, prescription drugs and even arsenic. And, be cautious about bottled water. Approximately 40% of all bottled water is actually tap water in a bottle.

Best choices? I suggest Reverse Osmosis or Distilled. Both of these kinds of water are filtered and have all toxins removed. With that being said, you must appreciate that these water filtration systems remove all harmful contaminants, AND all minerals too. So, you must put the minerals back in. Simply add a pinch of Himalayan or Celtic Unprocessed Sea Salt to your water.

Is it good to drink water while eating?

No. Drinking water during meals may dilute your digestives enzymes and stomach acids, and this makes the breaking down of food less effective. Drinking water while eating can also lead to sagging or heaviness in the stomach as well as drowsiness. If you must have something to drink while eating, small sips of warm water is best.

Micronutrients:

Vitamins and minerals are found in all natural foods and are needed by our bodies to maintain health and function.

Minerals

Minerals play different roles, some of which include aiding the production and functioning of hormones and enzymes, working as constituents of teeth and bones, and regulating bodily fluids. Calcium, Magnesium, Potassium, Sodium, Iron, Zinc and Chromium are some examples of minerals.

Vitamins

Vitamins are organic compounds. This means they have carbon atoms- as opposed to minerals, which are purely inorganic in nature. While vitamins are unstable during food processing, preparation, and cooking, minerals are more stable when it comes to food preparation.

Vitamins play an important role in the sustenance of life, and while some are produced in our bodies, others are not. Vitamins help in the prevention and treatment of a number of medical conditions. (High cholesterol, heart disease, skin and eye disorders to name a few.)

Vitamins are either fat soluble (disperse and are stored in fat) or water soluble (dissolve in water). Your body is able to store fat soluble vitamins in fat tissues, while water soluble vitamins are expelled through your body more quickly. As a result, replenishing water soluble vitamins is required more frequently. Fat soluble vitamins comprise of vitamins A, D, E, & K; Vitamins B complex and C fall under water soluble vitamins.

Q & A

Does a varied diet get enough vitamins and minerals?

I believe that prior to 1950- Yes, we could get all vitamins/minerals we needed from our food. Unfortunately, with today's commercial farming, I am sorry to say- No, I don't believe any diet (organic, farm grown, or commercially farmed) will give enough necessary vitamins/minerals for many reasons including a lack of field rotation/growth hormones/GMO seeds/sedentary raised animals.

Do we need to take supplements to get our necessary vitamins and minerals?

Yes we do, and for the following reasons.

- In the Standard American Diet (SAD diet) most consume refined, processed, boxed or canned foods that have lost most of its original nutrients during the processing.
- Nutrients are lost from the time the food is picked until it is eaten. Fresh fruit and veggies are picked early, ripen during travel, and sit on a shelf waiting to bought, then sit in fridge or counter, then are cooked then eaten. So many nutrients are lost during this process.
- Crops are grown in fields that have not been rotated allowing for mineral replenishment in soil. Our plants do not contain the nutrients they did decades ago.
- Our animals are fed poor quality foods, toxic foods and become toxic. We are what we eat. Nutrient deficient animals or plants means nutrients deficient food for us.

How do we choose the best vitamin and mineral that is suited to each individual?

Choose a natural plant source, not synthetic or man made source.

Liquid and powder are absorbed faster than capsules and tablets and are easier to take for those who have difficulty swallowing pills. Capsules are better absorbed than tablets (some tablets have a coating that prevents absorption) and are often not taken consistently as most have difficulty swallowing.

My favourite is called Vemma. It is a liquid multi vitamin/mineral containing 12 full spectrum vitamins and 65 plant sourced minerals. Two ounces taken daily is suggested. You can order Vemma at www.andreathatcher.vemma.com. Vemma is simple, convenient and complete.

What are the best sources of calcium?

Contrary to popular belief, dairy is NOT a good source of calcium. The best sources for calcium include:
- Unprocessed Himalayan or Celtic Sea Salt
- Green Leafy Veggies
- Sesame seeds
- Almonds or make your own almond milk
- Salmon (wild, not farmed)
- Sardines
- Soups made with broth from bones

WHAT YOU SHOULD KNOW ABOUT CALORIES

Is there a basic calories-per-day guideline for men/women?

No. Your required calorie intake is dependent on your metabolism, activity and current exercise level. It varies day to day, and it increases while under stress, and also increases with activity. As a baseline to build from, I don't believe a woman will get the necessary nutrients from a calorie restrictive diet below 1500-1800 calories and for a man below 2200-2500. Again, this is entirely dependent on many individual factors.

A general rule-of-thumb to follow is - eat when hungry. Stop when not. Don't eat till you feel full. DON'T eat because you're bored, or lonely. Your body never lies. It will not tell you it is hungry when it's not. We need to determine the difference between being thirsty, hungry, bored, lonely or simply out of habit.

If you are overweight, you are eating too many calories for your needs (boredom, loneliness, comfort, enjoyment, etc). If you are underweight, you are not eating enough. Calorie counting is INEFFECTIVE for finding your healthy weight. Listening to your body and its physical needs is the answer.

How many calories do I need and how many calories do I burn?

How many calories you burn, again, depends on your body make up, your daily activity levels and the amount of exercise you do.

Here's an example of how to calculate your needs:

Step 1

Determine Basal Metabolic Rate by multiplying body weight by 10 calories (BMR)_____

Step 2

Determine Daily Activity Rate (DAR) _____
Multiply BMR by percentage of activity level
_____X_____ = _____

Sedentaryadd 20 to 40%
Moderately Active add 40 to 60%
Very Activeadd 60 to 80%

A sedentary lifestyle implies that you are not active regularly; for example a computer programmer that spends most of the day sitting. If you take long walks, keep yourself moving through the day in a profession such as a store clerk, you have light activity levels. Exercising regularly and rarely sitting while working like a waitress or a nurse would put you in the moderate activity level bracket; and athletes, personal trainers and physical labourers like construction workers fall under the very active category.

Step 3

Determine Average Exercise Rate(add together) _____

Cardio: _____calories burned
Resistance: _____calories burned

Step 4

Determine Actual Daily Caloric Requirement by adding steps 1, 2 and 3. _____

Q & A

Is a calorie a calorie regardless of where it comes from (calorie from chocolate cake vs. chicken breast)?

No.
Calories from live, natural foods provide calories and nutrients the body needs; whereas 'empty' calories i.e. sugar, cake, cookies, chocolate, etc, contain calories with NO nutrients (we call these anti nutrient foods).

For example, 1500 calories a day from twinkies (anti nutrient) vs. 1500 calories a day from whole natural foods will have completely different responses. Anti nutrients break our bodies down, causing stress, weight gain and poor health. Nutrient rich foods build our body up, leading to greater health, vitality, energy, clarity and healthy weight.

How can one calorie differ from another?

This can easily be explained through an example using sugar. For instance, while both fructose and glucose can work in providing you with the same number of calories, the way they are metabolized is rather different. Glucose is used directly by the cells of our bodies. It needs no special processing. Fructose, you should know, actually works in tricking your body's appetite control system, and can thereby lead to weight gain.

This is because fructose presence suppresses your hunger hormone called ghrelin and does nothing to stimulate the hormone which controls satiety or fullness, called leptin. This can lead to various problems including elevated cholestorol, weight gain, obesity, high blood pressure, and in time, insulin resistance. If not regulated, fructose intake can impact the body's insulin levels in a negative manner as well as the way it is processed, and bear in mind that insulin plays an important role in regulating fat within the body.

So in this example, two kinds of sugars with the same number of calories are metabolised by your body differently and elicit a different response from your body.

NOTES:

UNDERSTANDING AN INGREDIENT LABEL

Nutrition Facts

Serving Size 1 cup (228g)
Servings Per Container about 2

Amount Per Serving

Calories 250   Calories from Fat 110

	% Daily Value*
Total Fat 12g	18%
Saturated Fat 3g	15%
Trans Fat 3g	
Cholesterol 30mg	10%
Sodium 470mg	20%
Total Carbohydrate 31g	10%
Dietary Fiber 0g	0%
Sugars 5g	
Proteins 5g	

Vitamin A	4%
Vitamin C	2%
Calcium	20%
Iron	4%

* Percent Daily Values are based on a 2,000 calorie diet.
Your Daily Values may be higher or lower depending on
your calorie needs:

	Calories:	2,000	2,500
Total Fat	Less than	65g	80g
Saturated Fat	Less than	20g	25g
Cholesterol	Less than	300mg	300mg
Sodium	Less than	2,400mg	2,400mg
Total Carbohydrate		300g	375g
Dietary Fiber		25g	30g

For educational purposes only. This label does not meet the labeling
requirements described in 21 CFR 101.9.

How to read an ingredient label

An ingredient label comes with different kinds of information, and understanding the various aspects will definitely help you understand what you are eating.

- **Servings**: This will tell you how many servings are part of the product and just how much each serving weighs. Paying attention to this aspect is crucial as this affects all other counts as well. For instance, if a package comes with 4 half cup servings, and you end up eating the entire contents in one go, you are, in effect, consuming 4 servings.
  - **Calories**: This not only tells you the total calories (per serving), it also tells you how many calories are derived from fat, carbohydrate and protein.
  - **Percentage of daily value:** The '%Daily Value' or '%DVs' indicate how much of each ingredient you require on a daily basis (in order to prevent disease, not necessarily to be healthy), and these are based on a 2000 calorie diet (that is, a diet plan of 2000 calories per day).

Understanding Calories:

Looking at a label you will see the total calories per serving is 250.

Knowing that 1 gram of carbohydrate contains 4 calories, one gram of protein contains 4 calories and one gram of fat contains 9 calories, we see that:

- 108 calories come from fat (12 grams of fat x 9 calories per gram = 108 calories from fat)
- 124 calories comes from carbohydrate (31 grams of carbohydrate x 4 calories per gram = 124 calories from carbohydrate)

- 20 calories comes from protein (5 grams of protein x 4 calories per gram = 20 calories from protein)

Here are some common terms listed on labels as well—and what they really mean:

Low in Fat	This food has 3 grams or less of fat per serving. The reality – if nature made the food with fat, then the fat should be there. It doesn't matter if a food is low in fat or not - if it's a natural food.
Fat Free	This food has a fat amount so small health experts consider it nutritionally insignificant. The reality – again, if nature made the food as fat free then that is how we should be eating it. If it is a high fat food that man made fat free through chemical processing, then this is not healthy for us.
Cholesterol Free	This food contains less than 2 mg cholesterol. The Reality – the amount of cholesterol that you consume has a smaller effect than the amount of fat you consume. To keep your cholesterol level in a healthy range, you must keep your diet lower in both saturated fat and cholesterol.
Light	In Canada, the term 'light' must be followed by the attribute that is light. In the US, there is no regulation for using the term 'light'. Light could refer to color, texture, amount of sodium, fat, calories, or even flavour. This term could be misleading to some.

Ingredient List
Ingredients in the food are listed by weight from most to least. The ingredient list is a source of information for people with allergies or for people who avoid certain ingredients based on their beliefs. Educate yourself on what ingredients are. For example, anything ending in 'ose' is a form of sugar – fructose, lactose. Further, if you cannot pronounce the ingredient, it may be chemically based and not the most nutritious food choice for you.

When you next go grocery shopping, take the time to read labels and educate yourself on what you are eating. Is the food natural? How many chemicals are in the food? Is there Trans Fats in the food?

Also remember nutritional value. Just because a Boston Cream Donut has the caloric value of a snack and contains less than 30% calories from fat, does not mean it is a nutritious choice. It is high in sugar and unhealthy transfat, and low in necessary vitamins and minerals.

Q & A

What are food additives?

Any ingredient that is added to a food product while it is being processed/produced in order to enhance its taste/appearance or act as a preservative is referred to as a food additive. Salt and vinegar are two common food additives found in most kitchens. Others include:

- Food acids like lactic acid, citric acid, malic acid, etc.
- Nitrites and nitrates
- Artificial sweeteners
- Antibiotics (given to 'food producing' livestock)
- Preservatives like sulphites, sorbic acid, benzoic acid, etc.
- Stabilizers like agar

Food additives should definitely be avoided. People who are lactose intolerant should pay particular attention to lactose being used as an additive, as its use is common.

Other food additives you should avoid include:
- MSG (monosodium glutamate)
- Nitrites and Nitrates
- Caffeine

What does concentrate mean (as in 'concentrate juice)?

If a juice is made using a concentrate, it means that the volume of the juice has been reduced by removing the water content to a desired level for packaging, and the volume is gained back upon adding water. However, the process that is carried out to make the concentrate does more than remove the water content, and concentrates are known to deplete the juice's original nutritive value.

Understanding Sugar and Sugar on Your Labels

Limiting sugar intake is important if you are hoping to live a healthy life. What you should know is that sugar finds it way into our diets through a myriad of packaged, processed, or canned foods, as well as through salad dressings, processed meats, condiments, breakfast cereals, beverages, etc. Your overall intake of sugar should ideally remain under 6 teaspoons per day (around 25 grams).

There are different types of sugars and the roles they play also vary. Given below are the common types of sugar we encounter on a day to day basis:

- **Fructose**: Commonly extracted from corn, it comes with a low glycemic index (the rate that sugar from the food is absorbed by your body) although it does work in increasing insulin's secretion in the pancreas. It occurs naturally in most fruits, and since fruits are good sources of fibre, minerals, and vitamins, looking at them to get your quota of fructose is a good idea. Two to three servings of fruits per day is ideal, and limiting your fructose intake to around 25 grams is suggested if weight loss is your goal.

- **HFCS (High Fructose Corn Syrup):** Derived mostly from genetically modified corn, this form of sugar is cheaper and sweeter than its cane derived counterpart, and is easily the most common type of sugar to be used in the food industry. In today's world, an average adult consumes around sixty three pounds of HFCS every year.

- **Agave Nectar:** A relatively new sweetener; although a number of 'claims' have been made in regards to agave being good for health, the fact remains that it is high fructose. In fact, its fructose levels are considerably higher in comparison to those in maple syrup or honey. Agave nectar comes with more than 90% fructose, which, to me, makes it even worse for your health than HFCS.

- **White Sugar:** Derived from cane or beet, this form of sugar is refined as well as bleached. This processed food gives you nothing in the form of nutrition, and since it is completely devoid of nutrients, it actually works in depleting your body's supply of vitamins and minerals.

- **Brown Sugar:** Also derived from cane or beet, brown sugar is not subjected to the bleaching process. Raw cane sugar is amongst the best alternatives when it comes to brown sugars, although there are various others as well. Also, since brown sugar is not refined, it works in retaining minerals, vitamins, and enzymes which are beneficial to the human body.

Hidden Sugars?

You probably already know of the common names of sugars and could include fructose, glucose, maltose, and sucrose. However, there are lots of others sugars and sweeteners that you should be aware of as well. The next time you're looking at a food label, watch out for these.

- Amasake
- Barley malt
- Barley malt syrup
- Brown rice syrup
- Cane juice
- Caramelized foods
- Carbitol
- Carmel coloring
- Concentrated fruit juice
- Corn sweetener
- Corn syrup
- Dextrin
- Dextrose
- Diglycerides
- Disaccharides
- D-tagalose
- Evaporated cane juice
- Fructooligosaccharides (FOS)
- Fructose
- Fruit juice concentrate
- Galactose
- Glucitol
- Glucoamine
- Gluconolactone
- Glucose
- Glucose polymers
- Glucose syrup
- Glycerides
- Glycerine
- Glycerol
- Glycol
- Hexitol
- High-fructose corn syrup
- Honey
- Inversol
- Isomalt

- Karo syrups
- Lactose
- Levulose
- Malitol
- Malt dextrin
- Malted barley
- Maltodextrins
- Maltodextrose
- Maltose
- Malts
- Mannitol
- Mannose
- Maple syrup
- Molasses
- Monoglycerides
- Monosaccarides
- Nectars
- Pentose
- Polydextrose
- Polyglycerides
- Raisin juice
- Raisin syrup
- Ribose rice syrup
- Rice malt
- Rice sweeteners
- Rice syrup solids
- Saccharides
- Sorbitol
- Sorghum
- Sucanet
- Sucrose
- Trisaccharides
- Turbinado sugar
- Xylitol
- Zylose

The Harmful Kind of Sugars:

Not all sugars are equally harmful - here are ones which cause the most amount of damage.

- **Aspartame**: Easily amongst the worst options when it comes to substituting sugar, it is also amongst the ones which are used most commonly because of the cost factor. Aspartame is made up of aspartic acid, methanol, phenylalanine, and amino acids, and is a known neurotoxin and carcinogenic substance. The methanol in aspartame is converted into formaldehyde, and this neurotoxin/carcinogenic substance bonds with DNA and accumulates within cells.

- Consequently, while your everyday intake of diet sodas will not result in cancer overnight, it could, in the long run, not only result in the condition but also its rapid growth. This is because aspartame can not only cause cancer but can also result in the rapid movement and growth of cancer cells.

- In addition, Aspartame also works as an excitotoxin in relation to nerve cells, which simply means that it can cause nerve cells to function in an overexcited state that causes them to die. Also, since the signs of neurodegenerative disorders such as Parkinson Disease and Multiple Sclerosis are quite similar to that of Aspartame toxicity, this condition is not really easy to diagnose.

- **Sucralose**: Sucralose was discovered in the process of scientists trying to create a new pesticide, and people with regular intake of sucralose based sweeteners often complain of problems like anxiety, allergies, nausea, moodiness, absentmindedness, itching, rashes, diarrhoea, and in some cases, even seizures. Research has gone on to show that sucralose can have a negative impact on the 'good' bacteria within the digestive tract, and can change the metabolic reactions of certain medicines.

- **Acesulfame K**: On food labels, this ingredient could be listed as Sunnett, Ace-K, Acesulfame K potassium, or just Acesulfame K. Commonly used to enhance flavour, this sweetener is around two hundred times sweeter than sucrose; and although it has been approved by the US FDA, long term studies surrounding its use have not yet been carried out. It contains methylene chloride, a known carcinogen, and can result in nausea, depression, headaches, kidney and liver problems to name a few.

- **Saccharine**: Amongst the oldest artificial sweeteners, it is bitter to taste, and is generally mixed with other sweeteners because of the same reason. The use of saccharin is banned in several nations owing to its increasing the risk of contracting bladder cancer, and other associated side effects including breathing problems, headaches, allergies, diarrhoea, muscle dysfunction, irritability and skin eruptions.

What you should know about such artificial sweeteners, is that while they come with a low glycemic index, and no sugar or calories, they can still work inducing insulin release. This, in the long run, will have an adverse effect on your pancreas and your body's metabolism, as well as your weight. These chemicals, in my opinion, aren't meant to be used by human beings at all.

Healthier Sweetening Options:

Yes, there are healthy options which can be used to add sweetness to foods, and these include the following.

- **Honey**: While honey is easily amongst the most healthy and natural form of sugar, the honey we commonly get is denaturized by being subjected to high temperatures which end up killing the naturally occurring friendly bacteria and enzymes. Honey is 55% fructose and 45% glucose, and the best kind of honey is unpasteurized, unfiltered, and raw. While its glucose-fructose ratio is similar to that of HFCS, raw honey also gives you antioxidants, vitamins, and minerals. Darker honey is believed to be richer in antioxidants.

- **Stevia**: This is a plant that is native to South Ameica, and its use as a sweetener has been around for centuries. It is approximately three hundred times sweeter in comparison to conventional sugar, and the fact that it comes with no reported toxicity or side effects make it my personal favourite sugar substitute.

- **Other forms of natural sugars include**- molasses, barley malt, brown rice syrup, and maple syrup. To retain their natural properties it is important that they should not be filtered, refined, or pasteurized.

Sugar Alcohol:

Sugar alcohols refer to a new breed of sweeteners referred to as polyols. Common examples include isomalt, xylitol, sorbitol, and maltitol. Some of these sweeteners are plant based and some are derived from starches and sugars. For instance, maltitol is derived from seaweed; and sorbitol, from corn syrup. Since the body cannot absorb these completely, they don't have too much of an impact on your blood sugar levels, and they have a low glycemic index and low caloric content.

Their use can commonly be seen in sugar-free chewing gums, and this is because they do not promote the decaying of teeth. Xylitol actually works in inhibiting the growth of bacteria in the oral cavity. The one drawback is that since these aren't completely absorbed by the body, they can end up fermenting within the intestines, leading to diarrhoea, bloating, or gas.

Health Effects of Sugar:

You probably already know that sugar has a negative impact on your body. It can play havoc on blood sugar levels leading to hypoglycemia and diabetes. It will also suppress your immune system. For your body to function at its optimum best, it requires just around one teaspoon of sugar within its blood supply at any given time; too little or too much can both cause problems.

If your intake of sugar is lower than it should be you could suffer from Hypoglycaemia. Symptoms may include headaches, insomnia, heart palpitations, shakiness, dizziness, fatigue, light-headedness, lack of energy, depression, mood swings, or cravings. In such a scenario, it is natural that you would crave sugar, since this is the quickest way to get your blood sugar levels up. When you eat sugar in some form, your blood sugar levels will go up and you could feel better for around an hour, but you will soon suffer from low blood sugar levels again, causing you to reach for high sugar foods once again.

High blood sugar levels, on the other hand also have an adverse effect on your entire body. Cells throughout your body, in the presence of too much sugar, end up becoming sticky; this condition is referred to as glycation. What it basically means is that every single process is slowed down, your metabolism becomes sluggish, your brain becomes slow, your arteries plug up, circulation and repair are impaired, there could be a hormonal imbalance, digestion can go to crap, and you can suffer from nerve damage. In really simply words, this means that you are aging at a much faster rate.

Q & A

Why do People Crave Sugar?

Sugar cravings could be an indication of a deficiency of the mineral chromium, and this could be because refined sugar works in stressing the pancreas and in depleting chromium levels within the body. Giving into these cravings will work in reducing chromium levels even more, leading to further cravings. You could crave sugar/sweets simply because of the 'pleasure' factor too. For instance, chocolate is believed to work in stimulating serotonin production, a chemical commonly referred to as the 'feel good' hormone.

Overgrowth of yeast is something else that can result in sugar cravings, and this condition is commonly referred to as candidaisis (Candida, a kind of yeast, can be found naturally in the human body). Factors like excessive sugar in your diet or exposure to antibiotics can cause this yeast to grow rapidly, resulting in severe fatigue and vaginal yeast infections. When the presence of this yeast grows beyond a certain point, it results in rather strong cravings for starchy and sweet foods.

Some say to eliminate or limit fruit intake because of the sugar content ...

Fruit is a whole food, the way Mother Nature intended. If she didn't want us to be eating the natural sugar in fruit, she wouldn't have made the fruit with sugar in it. I think it ridiculous to eliminate fruit because of the sugar content. Fruit contains a variety of essential vitamins and minerals and is a great source of fibre. Fruit is also a great source of energy and curbs cravings for crappy sugar found in chocolate bars and candy.

What is the Connection between Sugar and Weight Gain?

While your body does not need to process glucose in any way (as it is used by your cells directly) fructose must be processed by your liver. This metabolism of fructose is quite complicated, and its over-consumption leads to an increase in the production of fat. As this fat is not used for fuel in sedentary people, liver damage and fat deposits are common. Combine a high sugar diet with a sedentary lifestyle and weight gain results.

NOTES:

WEIGHT LOSS AND WEIGHT GAIN

Q & A

How does your body gain weight?

Your Basic Metabolic Rate (BMR) is the amount of energy or calories that your body requires at rest. Your BMR is determined by your lean weight – your muscle, organs, bones and tissues. You also need additional energy for daily activities at work and at home (Daily Activity Rate, or DAR), and for exercise (Average Exercise Rate, or AER). Your daily caloric requirement is a combination of the calories used by your BMR, your DAR and your AER. When you eat more calories than your body requires, you gain weight.

When you take in more food energy than your body needs, excess energy is stored as fat. (One pound of body fat is the equivalent of approximately 3500 calories of extra food energy). Body fat is concentrated energy for your body and has other main functions; it acts as a heat insulator, it cushions your organs, bones and joints and it is necessary for absorption of Vitamins A, D, E and K. For these reasons, having adequate body fat is important. However, excess fat can become a health risk to you and quite often has emotional implications as well.

According to the American Council on Exercise healthy ranges of body fat % for a man are 7-25% and for a woman are 15-33%. There is no real accurate way to take your actual body fat percentage. Common methods such as Bio-electrical Impedance and calipers used in most gyms can be 3-8% inaccurate when measuring.

2. How does your body lose weight?

The true purpose of dieting is not to lose weight but to lose FAT. When you begin a diet that causes rapid weight loss, the first "weight" that is lost is the water that is stored in your body. As a reaction to this dehydration, your body increases the production of anti-diuretic hormones, which result in your body storing even more water. Because 2 cups of water equals approximately one pound on the scale, you will eventually gain the weight back on the scale. Adequate hydration indicates your lean weight (muscle, bones, tissues and organs) should be approximately 70% water.

It's not just water that you lose when you diet and lose weight rapidly – it is also muscle. According to Dr. Michael Colgan – (on low calorie diets, meaning less than 1200 calories per day), up to 45% of weight lost is lean weight. Because the body is not taking in enough food energy to meet its demands, the body must burn stored energy for fuel. Unfortunately, it is not only fat that your body burns; it is also the tissue from your muscles and organs. Retaining muscle is essential for losing body fat because it is your lean weight which determines your metabolism: the less muscle you have the lower your Basal Metabolic Rate (BMR) is, and the harder it is to lose fat.

Diets that are low in calories and cause a rapid weight loss will cause your body to go into defensive action. Your body increases the production of the fat storing enzyme, making you more efficient at storing fat. Secondly, your body's metabolism slows down due to the loss of muscle. All of this leads to you gaining more weight, and gaining it faster than you did last time, the moment you stop dieting and return to real eating.

How does your body find its healthy weight?

The true purpose of weight reduction is to lose body fat while maintaining your muscle and body water. The formula is simple: expend more energy than you take in. In other words, reduce the amount of food you consume, and/or increase your activity level. For successful weight management, lose no more than half a pound to one pound of fat per week by reducing your required daily caloric intake by no more than 20%. These changes will not trigger your body's defence systems or lower your BMR. Exercise, managing your stress level and having a healthy attitude and body image is also extremely important for finding your healthy weight.

Is there really such a thing as nutrition for weight loss?

Yes. Portion control and balanced nutrition (protein, carbohydrates and fat in YOUR healthy ratio at each meal) will lead to your healthy weight, and NOT calorie restriction. Replace packaged, processed, pasteurized, refined foods with whole foods in their natural state. These foods contain nutrients your body recognizes and utilizes so you are less likely to eat empty calories that lead to weight gain. There are no specific foods or combinations of foods that will miraculously cause anyone to lose weight.

What is the best nutrition plan for energy and for fat loss?

Eat every 2 to 4 hours, and eat protein, carbohydrates, and fat at each meal/snack. Do not count calories, do not starve yourself, maintain portion control and eat till you are no longer hungry-NOT till you are full!!! This works for all, for any goal i.e. energy or fat loss.

What's wrong with Weight control diets?

Weight control diets, in this day and age, are a dime a dozen. All are designed for quick weight loss, and have little to no consideration for improving your health, or for the long term negative effects on your health; both physically and emotionally.

- **Low calorie diets:** A low calorie diet would involve your consuming foods which are low in calories (or no calories due to man made fake sugar like aspartame or sucralose) or consuming a low number of calories per day (lower than 1500 for a woman or 2200 for a man for example). A low calorie diet would not really focus on your consuming healthy foods; quick weight loss being the primary aim. Such diets can work in reducing pounds, although the results are generally short-term. Bottom line: Starvation ALWAYS works for weight loss. Anorexia is Free. No point in spending thousands of dollars to join a company offering to teach you how to lose weight through caloric restriction. With a reduction in calories comes a reduction in nutrients. With a reduction of nutrients comes a reduction in health. Are you prepared to forfeit your health for rapid weight loss? We all know Anorexia is unhealthy. Are you aware that ALL calorie restriction diets are leading you toward Anorexia?

- **Low fat diets:** Around 30% of the calories required by the body to function should come through fats in a healthy diet, and this is something that is overlooked in following a low fat diet. A low fat or a fat free diet does not give the body enough fat soluble vitamins and essential fatty acids, and while it can result in short term weight loss, it can also lead to various problems in the long run. You should, however, avoid trans fats as these are man made and work in raising the body's 'bad' cholesterol.

- **Detox diets:** The basic premise behind these diets is to detoxify the body by getting rid of the body's toxins while providing increased energy, better skin, and even weight loss. How well they work though is another matter altogether. Detox diets work by eliminating various foods from your diet, and these could include sugar, dairy products, grains, processed foods and the like. In some instances, you would be asked to go on an entirely liquid diet or a limited diet with a series of pills to take. Most detox diets do away with providing important nutrients and this can have less than desirable effects. For example, the body can start destroying muscle tissues to get the energy it requires.

- A detox diet could be required for people who suffer from illnesses, and shouldn't be chosen from a magazine. See a Naturopathic Doctor or Nutritionist who will advise you on the best and healthiest detox diet for your specific needs.

Eating and Exercising

Q & A

What are the best after workout meals?

Any meal in your correct ratio of protein to carbohydrate to fats, (start with 50% from Carbohydrates, 25% from Fats and 25% from Protein) that contains your favourite healthy carbohydrates to re-fuel, protein to repair and rebuild, and fat for fullness, is good after a workout.

What is the best protein to have before and after a workout?

This varies for different people. The one your body tolerates best both before and after a workout is best for you. If you are unsure, simply track the foods you eat both before and after a workout and track your responses. Over time you'll learn what works best for your individual needs.

 For some the best protein will be non-meat sources such as beans and rice, or quinoa. For others it could be eggs, fish, red meat, or poultry. For others, a protein shake works best as it is blended and easier for some to digest.

Very little protein (as much as an egg for example) tends to be enough before a workout. Larger amounts of protein are best taken post workout to allow your body to repair and rebuild.

What are fast energy foods?

Carbohydrates! Fast energy from fruit or fruit juices and longer release energy from whole grain sources such as rice or quinoa, or from starchy veggie such as potato or squash.

Do I need extra protein if I'm exercising?

If you are exercising, you'll need more overall calories including more protein, more fat and more carbohydrate. Once you've calculated your caloric needs, (See page 60 to Calculate your caloric needs) start with 50% of your diet coming from carbohydrate, 25% from fats and 25% from protein. As you learn how your body responds to exercise and this ratio of food intake, you'll be able to increase or decrease your need for protein based on how you feel, not based on a number randomly chosen because it worked for someone else. The only way to know what works for you is to track your food intake and how your body responds.

NOTES:

WORKING TOWARDS A HEALTHY DIET

Q & A

What are some of the healthier diet plans out there?

If you look for different diet plans, you'll probably be surprised by the number of results thrown your way. All diet plans incorporate certain foods and do away with certain others, and given below are some of the most prevalent diet plans you'll come across.

Vegan: A vegan eats only plant based foods and refuse to consume any food from an animal source, be it meat, eggs, fish, or any form of dairy (milk, cheese or yogurt). Vegans also abstain from consuming processed or cooked foods which come with animal derived constituents like gelatine or rennet for example. I don't agree with Vegan as a way of eating. Vitamin B-12 must be supplemented as it cannot be obtained from a Vegan diet.

Vitamin B12 is found in animal products. If one eliminates all forms of animal products then one must supplement (a man made product) Vitamin B12 for good health. However, I think if Mother Nature intended us to be vegan, she would have put B12 in a plant source too instead of animal sources. I believe we are supposed to eat meat, only the ratio of meat to carbohydrates to fat is very individual. Some require more meat, others less.

Vegetarianism: There are different classifications of Vegetarianism:
- Lacto-vegetarian: Will eat dairy products
- Lacto-ovo-vegetarian: Will eat dairy products, as well as eggs
- Pesco vegetarian: Will eat fish
- Pollo- vegetarian: Will eat chicken
- One can be a lacto, ovo, pesco, pollo vegetarian which means they eat everything but red meat
- One can be any variation of the above (except Vegan which is NO animal source)

Raw Food Diet: A raw foods diet consists of unprocessed raw vegan foods that have not been heated above115 degrees Fahrenheit (46 degrees Celsius). It is believed that foods cooked above this temperature have lost their enzymes and thus a significant amount of their nutritional value and are harmful to the body, whereas uncooked foods provide living enzymes and proper nutrition.

This can be very challenging to maintain, although the health benefits of raw food eating are well documented. Most will experience increase in energy, better bowel movements, deeper and more restful sleep, improved skin, hair and nails, and an overall felling of well being.

What are eating disorders?

Eating disorders include a number of medical conditions caused by of the lack of, or excessive intake of food, or because of unusual eating habits. These can not only have an impact on the sufferer's physical health, but mental health as well. Given below are some of the most common eating disorders.

Anorexia Nervosa

- Restricting food to the point of losing 15% of normal weight
- In women – the loss of 3 consecutive menstrual cycles
- Denying seriousness of low body weight
- Great fear of gaining weight and becoming fat
- Affects 1% of society with 90% being women
- Only mental illness that can cause death

Bulimia Nervosa

- Eating large amounts of food with a feeling of loss of control 2 or more times per week for at approximately 3 months
- Extreme measures taken to compensate for binge episodes such as purging by vomiting, over exercise, diuretics or laxatives
- Affects approximately 5-6% of society (many are males)
- Usually of normal weight

Binge Eating Disorder

- Still being researched
- Binge Eating 2 or more times per week for at least 6 months
- Feeling of loss of control while eating
- Eating alone due to embarrassment, guilt or feeling bad about oneself
- More likely to be obese or overweight

What are the common food deficiencies?

Food deficiencies account for the most common form of nutritional disorders and their risk is most pronounced during one's formative years - adolescence in particular. Reasons attributed to this include poor dietary choices, fast lifestyles, and quick growth. Here are some examples:

Magnesium: Magnesium deficiency can lead to confusion, anxiety, nervousness, insomnia, restlessness, depression, heart palpitations, heart attacks, weakness, constipation. Good sources of magnesium include seeds, beans, and green leafy vegetables.

Calcium: Deficiency in calcium can lead to weak bones, muscle cramps & weakness, and quicker tooth decay. Good sources of calcium include raw dairy products, green leafy vegetables, almonds, figs, and beans.

Zinc: Deficiency in Zinc can lead to ADD/ADHD, depression, irritability, memory impairment, paranoia, acne, hair loss, impotence, male infertility, lethargy, psoriasis, night blindness. Good sources of Zinc include beef, calf's liver, green peas, spinach, and mushrooms.

Vitamin D: Deficiency in Vitamin D can lead to an increased risk of cancer, diabetes, MS, Heart Disease, inflammation, chronic pain, cold/flu. Good sources of Vitamin D – The sun! 15-30 minutes a day of sun exposure without sunscreen (being careful not to burn) in the middle of the day. Best food choices are organ meats and eggs. If choosing Vitamin D in supplement form, choose the animal sourced D3 as it is more bio available for your body to use than the plant sourced Vitamin D2.

Essential Fatty Acids: While it might be hard to believe, there are a number of people who suffer from a deficiency in essential fatty acids. Deficiency in essential fatty acids can lead to an increased risk of anxiety & depression, dry skin, hair loss, easy bruising, repeated infections, etc. Good sources of essential fatty acids includes nuts, seeds like sunflower, pumpkin & flax, and oily fish such as salmon.

What is the best way to cleanse the body?

The simplest way to cleanse the body is to hydrate, lubricate and bulk - drink lots of purified water, eat healthy fats, and eat fibre - all from a certified organic source. Eliminate all foods that are not from Mother Nature (all in box/can/jar/package).

Also, bear in mind the following.

- Most store bought 'cleanses' are irritants to your system and cause you to poop a lot so you think it is working. We want to 'stimulate' not 'irritate' bowel movements.
- By regulating your digestive system, the body poops more, and this is one step in the cleansing process.
- There are different cleansing approaches to reducing digestive stress, restoring proper digestion and allowing for proper elimination and cleansing.
- See a Naturopathic Doctor or Natural Nutritionist to determine the best cleanse for you.

What is food combining and is it important for digestion or a gimmick?

The food combining concept is used to promote better digestive health, by reducing stress/energy required to digest. Different enzymes break down different foods and different foods break down at different rates, i.e. fruit is digested quickly and meat slowly. When eaten together, the fruit gets 'stuck' while the meat is digesting. This may lead to bloating and gas. Bear in mind the following:

- Always eat fruit alone (especially melon as it is the fastest to digest)
- Eat starches and veggies together
- Eat meat with non starchy veggies together
- Do not eat starches (bread, pasta, potato and rice) with proteins (meat)

What should you keep in mind while shopping for groceries?

If you do not know how to read food ingredient labels, it is important that you learn how to do so, because these will tell you just what the product in question comes with. These include aspects like serving size, number of servings, ingredients, calories contained, whether it is organic or not, etc.

Shopping for groceries also requires that you plan ahead of time and consider aspects such as how often you cook, how much time you devote to the process, and what you wish to eat in the coming days. Also important is that you make a list and ensure that you stick to it. Going to shop for groceries on an empty stomach is a definite no. The best way for you to eat healthy meals and snacks is to always have them ready to grab from your pantry and fridge. This means planning your meals ahead of time, as well as having a stock pile of healthy options in your kitchen.

Make sure you add fresh fruits and vegetables to your list, and try to avoid canned alternatives. In getting your quota of protein, add lean meats, fish (like whitefish or salmon), and legumes (like kidney beans or black beans), and lentils to your list. When it comes to buying grains, choose oats, quinoa or rice for example.

If you must buy processed foods, you should ideally look for food products with simple ingredients, and if you come across ingredients you cannot pronounce, don't eat them, or put the food in your '20% for the day'. In addition, steer clear of products which come with preservatives, artificial colour & flavours, hydrogenated oils, etc.

Remember when you go to the grocery store, to walk the perimeter of the store. Produce and Meat are all on the outside of the aisles. Only go into the aisles if you need spices or condiments, paper towels or toilet paper.

Choose Organic food options whenever possible.

Here are some helpful hints for your grocery shopping trip:

1. Plan Ahead. Use your Menu Planner to decide what meals and snacks you will have the next few days or a week.
2. Use your Menu Planner to create your grocery list.
3. Choose Certified Organic or Free Range whenever possible.
4. Shop at your local farmers market and purchase produce that is in season.
5. Always eat before going grocery shopping. You will purchase far less and far healthier groceries if you aren't hungry.
6. If preparation time is an issue, purchase pre-cut vegetables.
7. Keep a stock pile of frozen vegetables, meat and other staples in your freezer and replenish weekly.

GRAINS	FRUITS
Brown Rice/Wild Rice Sprouted Grain Breads/ Bagels/wraps (made without flour) Oats Quinoa	Domestic is best. Apples, Peaches, Pears, Plums, Berries Variety of colors, fresh or frozen
VEGETABLES	**MILK PRODUCTS***
Green is best. Spinach, Romaine, Kale, Bok Choy, Cucumbers, Peppers, Asparagus, Broccoli, Brussel Sprouts, Artichoke, Cabbage, Celery, Turnip Greens, Zucchini Variety of colors, fresh or frozen	Rice, Almond, Potato Milk Raw Organic Cheese Raw Plain Yogurt Butter *Raw, Organic cheese is available in most grocery stores in Canada. Raw milk, or yogurt can be purchased from a farmer that sells raw dairy products.

MEAT AND ALTERNATIVES	SPICES AND SEASONINGS
Beef, Pork, Chicken, Turkey, Fish, Wild Game Beans, Lentils, Chick Peas Free Range or Organic Eggs Raw Nuts and Seeds Raw or Natural Nut Butter	Salt, pepper, oregano, cumin, tarragon, chili powder etc. Fresh Garlic and Ginger Olive Oil, Vinegars (balsamic, raspberry etc)

CONDIMENTS AND OTHER
Pickles, ketchup, mustard, relish, mayonnaise, jelly, spreads, coffee, tea, hot chocolate, soup broth etc.

What foods should I eat for nice hair and nails?

Fats and proteins! Fats should come through sources like fish, flax, nuts, seeds, avocado, green leafy vegetables; and proteins from meat, fish, eggs (proteins help the body to repair and rebuild).

Are there foods which cause excessive bloating/gas?

Typically, the foods that cause bloating or gas are the ones you shouldn't be eating. Your body is telling you that it cannot break down the foods you ate, so the best thing you can do is stop eating them.

Common foods that cause bloating or gas:

Dairy
Gluten
Eggs
Shellfish
Soy
Corn
Protein powders
Processed foods
Refined or sugary foods

Another cause of gas/bloating is eating a large amount of fibre in a single sitting. If you are not accustomed to eating a lot of fibre, introduce it into your daily diet over time.

If you are not used to eating veggies or a lot of fiber, remember that in the beginning it will cause you bloating and gas if you over do it. Take your time and increase your fibre a bit each day until you reach 25-40 grams.

What foods should Blood Pressure patients avoid?

People who suffer from high blood pressure should limit their intake of salt, alcohol, fatty foods and caffeine.
- Alcohol has a direct relation with raising blood pressure, and also plays a role in damaging blood vessel walls.
- Salt intake leads to the kidney retaining excessive fluids, thereby resulting in increased blood pressure.
- Trans fats /fried foods have an adverse effect on blood vessels as well as the heart.
- The effect on caffeine of high blood pressure seems to vary case by case and depends on factors like drinking habits, the volume consumed on an ongoing basis, pre-existence of the condition, etc.

While similar restrictions aren't placed on people who suffer from low blood pressure (except limiting the intake of alcohol), they are asked to make some dietary changes as well.

- They are advised to increase their intake of sodium.
- They are advised to eat small meals which are low in carbohydrates at regular intervals.
- Increase fluid intake, preferably in the form of water.
- Some people, given their tolerance to caffeine, are also asked to increase their caffeine intake.

Is drinking wine good for the heart?

No. Alcohol is a toxic poison that must be filtered by the liver. It is linked to cancer, migranes and weight gain to name a few problems related to drinking.

Red wine has been cited as being good for your heart because wine contains resveratrol, melatonin and flavonoids, all of which are good for you.

Flavonoids have antioxidant properties.
Melatonin thought to reduce inflammation
Resveratrol helps lower blood pressure, and is an antioxidant and anti inflammatory

Don't be fooled. Alcohol, even wine is harmful to your health.

NOTES:

Eating Habits

Q & A

If someone has poor eating habits, is it better to change over time or should the change to healthy be all at once?

This, too, depends on personality type, and there is no right or wrong way to do it. I personally prefer to make changes over time, as for my personality it leads to greater success. Choose the way that leads to your long term success. No one knows you better then you. Take the path you believe you will stick to for the long term.

How can I get my whole family eating clean?

Start by following the age old adage, "become the change you want to see." It is important that you lead by example. Do it for yourself and your family will support you and want to get involved. Educate them on the harmful effects of commercial foods and why you made the decision to eat clean. Tell them how eating clean will improve and help each family member reach his/her own personal goal. Don't do what most do – by preaching to them and forcing them to change at your rate. This is your journey not theirs. So respect that, and in turn they will want to join your journey when they are ready – not when you tell them they should.
And make it fun.

CONCLUSION

Learning about health and nutrition and not taking action is of no use. The information in this book combined with consistent (80% of the time!) action, will have a positive and lasting effect on your health and well being.

Remember, if you do what you've always done, you'll get what you've always gotten. In order to see change, you need to change. Decide. Right now. Take at least one suggestion made in this book and decide that you will implement that change today. Right now.

Living a healthy, vibrant, energetic life is simple. It's a choice. One you get to make each day. Making healthy food choices may not always be convenient. It may not always be easy. It may not always be what you want in the moment. But, it's worth it. The other option is to be overweight, tired, and suffering from illness and disease.

Live 80/20, and eat the way Nature intended. Success will be yours.

In health,
Andrea

SUCCESS STORIES

From Karen Smith...

"Andrea, you are an amazing coach, instructor, and role model for me. I have learned many things while taking your courses, including how to manage my IBS. You, suggested trying to go off gluten and dairy at the same time, and I thought that would be impossible. With perseverance and determination I have been off both for three months and because of it, I simply feel far better. Like everyone, I occasionally cheat from my dietary regiment, and when I do my IBS flares up which reminds me why I shouldn't.

Surprisingly, I don't really miss bread anymore, though I do eat gluten free bread once in awhile. You also talked about the importance of cutting out sugar and processed foods. This seemed nearly impossible, but with a little planning and determination I made it happen. My husband and children don't eat exactly the same way I do, and their snacks create temptations for me to avoid. In those rare times where I do eat processed or sugary foods, it's only a matter of hours before I feel downright awful again.

Andrea, before your advice, I thought it impossible to eat oatmeal without sugar; now days I wouldn't even dream about adding any. My cravings for simple sugars have disappeared, and I love how oatmeal tastes now with flax and chia added instead.

My whole life, I have always been very active, but not as diligent when it came to healthy eating. Food was my biggest obstacle, but if I can do this, I believe anyone can.

Thank you Andrea for your priceless wisdom and how it's helped me feel better than I have in a long time."

From Kristi Czank...

"Taking your nutrition course changed my life. In 2009 my body was in shock from months of starvation and fat burners after my fitness competition. I then immediately gained more weight than I knew what to do with. I didn't understand the relationship between the food I was eating and why my body was reacting the way it was. Andrea, you mapped it out. First, you helped me to understand my personal relationship with food and how that played a role in my life. You then lead me on a journey that opened my eyes to appreciate what my body required in order to be the best and healthiest it could be. I learnt every dynamic of nutrition including why, when, what and how it could work with me instead of against me.

What I have obtained from this course is invaluable. Two years later, my own body and mind transformation continues to serve as a reminder of this. I am in full control of my healthy lifestyle and because I know better, I do better.

With everything in me I thank you Andrea for this information. You are steadfast in your beliefs about natural nutrition and you have given me all the tools I need to succeed.

This information needs to be brought to the attention of high schools and young emerging athletes and coaches."

From Shelby Douglas...

"Working with you is truly a life-changing experience. I was dealing with a variety of health issues from stress and anxiety to managing fatigue and chronic sinusitis. You were very thorough in looking at all areas of my life to determine how to not only to improve my diet and health but how my diet would affect all the health concerns I had. You are so knowledgeable in understanding how our diet and the foods we eat play a major role in our health and overall well-being. You were able to pin-point what foods I should avoid and which foods I should eat and your suggestions and meal plans were easy and simple to follow. I have worked with doctors and naturopaths but it wasn't until I started seeing you that my overall health begin to change. I am less stressed and anxious, have little or no fatigue, sleep better at night and haven't had any sinus infections (I used to get 3 a year). Andrea, you truly know how to keep the body strong and healthy and I have recommended you to all my family and friends."

Andrea Thatcher,

Registered Holistic Nutritionist, (RHN)

www.AndreaThatcher.com